COLOUR HEALING

Psychologically we are all affected by colour.
This book explains a revolutionary new method
of healing by which the rays of coloured lamps
are applied to diseased organs of the body, with
amazingly beneficial results.

D063150D

By the same author
PALMISTRY
    Your Destiny in Your Hands
NUMEROLOGY
    The Secret Power of Numbers

COLOUR HEALING

Chromotherapy and How it Works

by

MARY ANDERSON

THE AQUARIAN PRESS
Wellingborough, Northamptonshire

First published 1975
Second Edition (completely revised, enlarged and reset) 1979
Second Impression 1980
Third Impression 1981

© MARY ANDERSON 1979

This book is sold subject to the condition that it shall not, by way of trade or otherwise, be lent, re-sold, hired out, or otherwise circulated without the publisher's prior consent in any form of binding or cover other than that in which it is published and without a similar condition including this condition being imposed on the subsequent purchaser.

ISBN 0 85030 170 X

Printed and bound in Great Britain by
Richard Clay (The Chaucer Press) Ltd.,
Bungay, Suffolk.

CONTENTS

INTRODUCTION

Gradually, since the end of the war, colour has been coming back into our lives, taking up the place it held in Regency times after its long eclipse under the Victorians.

Contemporary colour is bold and bright, perhaps this is the defiant gesture of a frightened world where the Bomb looms large and our breakfast cornflakes take second place to each new horror revealed in newsprint, or perhaps it is that we are so uninhibited now. Whatever the reason, the new colours are here; browns, greys and creams have been ousted by bold, true colours. The reds are very red, the blues are exquisite, ranging from a very pale pastel blue to indigo, the greens delight and soothe us and the yellows are bold, having caught a little bit of sunshine on the way.

Colour expresses the way we think and then reacts back on us from our surroundings, either raising or lowering our spirits. It is evident that the richness and diversity of colour which we see around us at the present time reflects the thinking of a more joyful, open and honest age than the one just passed.

The fact that so much attention is now spent

on making homes tasteful and yet bright and easy to live in, shows that there is a general recognition of the important effect that colour has upon the personality. This is, of course, now directly recognized by the medical and hospital authorities, in that they seek to cheer the patients who are low by the use of reds, pinks and orange in their decorations, and to tranquillize those who are over-excited with all shades of blue and green.

Contemporary architecture helps as a background to the new taste in colour. It is far more difficult to show off contemporary furnishings to advantage in old-fashioned surroundings, although much ingenuity has been used in an endeavour to do just this. Coach houses, mews properties, and those gloomy abodes beloved of the Victorians, have been transformed by new ideas in colour.

When we touch on colour in dress, there has been a complete revolution, To prove this we need only say that *some* men are now wearing colours, if not for everyday office wear, at least at the weekends, the older ones a little shyly and the younger as to the manner born. As to women's clothes, these are nearly always bright. You only have to look up or down a busy shopping centre to see the little dots of colour moving to and fro amidst the grey sea of men.

Psychologically, of course, we are much affected by colour. We are cheered by vivid colours, while drab colours give us a correspondingly dull feeling. Red warms us. The warmth of an open fire is unexcelled, for although we can get a more even warmth through other forms of heating, the sight of the burning red coals affects us psychologically, and we associate a real home with a fire glowing there, ready and waiting for us to return. Even more friendly and warming is the heat given out by a peat or log fire, with its country associations, implying peace and security against the elements.

Blue is a cold colour, soothing to the eyes and mind alike. Green harmonizes us. If we wish to refresh ourselves we go to the countryside, where the green of nature restores us after the city has taken its toll of our nerves. As a mental stimulant, yellow is unbeaten and anyone who would like brilliant conversation in their drawing room (and who would not?), should first of all ask promising types and bear in mind that a good light yellow introduced somewhere in the room through the medium of the furnishings or the wall will be stimulating to the mental powers.

The sayings, 'Seeing red' and 'feeling blue', 'green with jealousy' and 'black with rage', all relate to actual changes which take place in the colours of our own electro-magnetic field due to changes in our emotions. This electro-magnetic field which surrounds everything, not only the human being, is often referred to as the aura. It is quite easy to assure yourself of the truth of this assertion by a little experiment. Ask a friend to stand with a light behind him and against a light-coloured wall. It is often easier to see the aura by not looking at it directly, but by concentrating on some point on the person's body, like the end of his nose – embarassing perhaps, so try his tie instead – then gradually you will see the faint glow around the head first and then around the whole body. To some people the aura appears to be white at first, but with practice, the colours will appear.

This aura, which is usually visible to sensitives, is often the means by which the colour healer diagnoses. The affected organ or part will show a dark or discoloured mark in the aura over the place where the disharmony exists. As each colour has a different vibration, colour healing is really operating on exactly similar lines to any other form of healing. In the same way that the doctor hopes that his pills will adjust the disharmony in the vibrational rate, so the contact or colour healer hopes for the same effect. The chemical imbalance of the body – which shows itself as a disease – may be corrected by chemical means or by means of the fine rays sent out in colour healing.

The colour healer having diagnosed by the condition, or in some instances having been told by the patient and checked this by his own observations, will proceed to apply remedial colours where there is a deficiency, or contrasting colours where there is an excess. He may do this by applying the rays of different coloured lamps or simply by directing the invisible rays which swirl around and through us day and night. He acts as a selector and conveyor of power, which he passes on to the patient. Some patients feel the application of the rays, others feel nothing, but all must benefit, although some more than others.

Taken all in all, colour is an integral part of our lives. It brings us joy, gaiety, and – when we need it – healing. Visible and invisible it affects us powerfully, for in it we live and have our being.

CHAPTER ONE

THE SCIENTIFIC BACKGROUND

We are all affected by colour in our everyday lives; but what is colour? The shortest definition which the dictionary gives us is that it is a quality of light. In an everyday sense we accept that our environment is subject to fluctuations in this quality of light, the day may be sunny, or drab and wet, and there are many variations in between these two poles. This is due to the rays or vibrations which are continually playing around and through everything in the world, although in most instances we cannot see them with our physical sight.

However, there is an inner significance behind the outer show and to the occultist and to many colour healers there is an age-old belief that in the truest sense *colour is life* and that the play of colour which manifests as light is the visible expression of the Divine mind, of the one life principle in the form of light waves.

The ancient Egyptians knew of the power and influence of colour and in their great temples, such as Karnak and Thebes, there were *colour halls* where research into the use of colour and colour healing was practised.

System of Colour Science

Manuscripts from these early times show that in India, China and Egypt, the healer priests had a complete system of colour science, based on the law of correspondence between the sevenfold nature of man and the sevenfold division of the solar spectrum. Therefore the fundamental laws and principles governing the cosmic energy we know as colour have always been present in the Ancient Wisdom teachings for the teachers and healers of all ages. However, modern research, physics, and metaphysics are all uncovering, as in many other fields, the wisdom of the ancients regarding the use of colour in healing, and we will view the matter first of all from the more orthodox angle, where doctors and scientists have interested themselves in research into the use of nature's finer forces, for the effective healing of many ailments, and as a result have actually used colour therapeutically with success.

Given that disease is a want of harmony in the system, the idea behind colour healing, or Chromotherapy, is to restore bodily imbalance through the application of beams of coloured light to the body.

Although colour healing, like many other sciences being revived today, bases its roots in the past, in modern times interest in it really began with experiments done on plants by Robert Hunt, whose book, *Researches on Light In Its Chemical Relations*, described the influences on plant growth of selected applications of light. The first book written on the use of colour for therapeutic purposes entitled *Blue and Red Light, or Light and Its Rays as Medicine*, by Dr S. Pancoast was published in 1877. Basically it dealt with the use of the stimulating red and the soothing blue rays, contrasting these in their effects on the human body.

The following year Dr E.D. Babbitt published his monumental work describing the effects of the different colours of the spectrum and their use as healing agents. However, it was a Hindu scientist by the name of D.P. Ghadiali who discovered the scientific principles which explain why and how the different coloured rays have various therapeutic effects on the organism. In 1933, after years of research Ghadiali published *The Spectro Chromemetry Encyclopaedia*, a master work on colour therapy. He worked and taught in the U.S.A., developing many types of colour lamps.

Ghadiali's Theories

The theories developed here come from Ghadiali's work. He stated that colours represent chemical potencies in higher octaves of vibration.

For each organism and system of the body there is a particular colour that stimulates and another that inhibits the work of that organ or system.

By knowing the action of the different colours upon the different organs and systems of the body, one can apply the correct colour that will tend to balance the action of any organ or system that has become abnormal in its functioning or condition.

The process of living in a healthy state involves a proper balance within the body of all the colour energies. When this balance is disturbed disease results, and if the imbalance becomes too great, death occurs. The aim of the science of colour healing is to combat disease by restoring the normal balance of colour energies within the body.

The earth and all its inhabitants obtain energy from the sun's rays – all elements known on earth are found in the sun, as shown by spectroscopic analysis. The sun's rays bring us the energies of every known element, from which all chemical combinations are made. White light contains the energies of all elements and chemicals found in the sun. The sun is constantly pouring white light energy into the atmosphere, thus 'charging' this atmosphere with the different types of energy necessary to sustain life.

The Auric Body

Man has an auric body surrounding and interpentrating his physical body. One of the functions of the aura is to absorb the white light energy from the atmosphere and split it into component colour energies, which then flow to the different parts of the body to vitalize them. Research indicates that it is probable that the effects noted from the use of colour therapy occur through the action of colour rays upon the auric body, which in turn influences the physical body.

In the human individual there are two basic processes at work all the time, namely anabolism and catabolism. The former is a building up and repairing process, while the latter is the opposite and deals with the elimination of toxic or waste products from the body. Good health can only be maintained if a proper balance is kept between the two processes of anabolism and catabolism, which together represent metabolism.

Primary Colours in Chromotherapy

Ghadiali found that the red ray is the colour of construction, that is, it maintains the number of red blood cells in the body and stimulates the liver, whilst the violet ray, which activates the spleen, is the colour of destruction or catabolism. He discovered that the spleen destroyed the older red blood cells and produced the white blood cells that combat bacteria.

In the spectrum, red – which stimulates the liver activity – is at one end of the visible spectrum of light, while violet – which stimulates splenic activity – is at the other end of the visible spectrum of light. The central or balancing colour of the spectrum of visible light is green, which is the colour that activates or encourages the activity of the pituitary gland, long known to be a master gland and controller of the other glands, and so affecting the action of every part of the body. Ghadiali said, 'we have come a long way, but we have now found our balancer for the body and it is green, the central body of the visible spectrum of light which fosters balance in the body between the opposing actions of the liver and the spleen, between anabolism and catabolism, and this is accomplished through the medium of the pituitary gland.'

From the foregoing it will be understood that Ghadiali found red, green and violet to be the primary colours in Chromotherapy. Red, yellow and blue, he said, were the primary colours when working with pigments, but light rays follow different laws from those that apply to the mixing of pigments. Ghadiali tested out many colour theories over decades, but these were the only ones proven right by extensive experiments.

You may ask: Why colour healing, when there are so many other methods? The answer is that Chromotherapy has many advantages. Ghadiali himself states, 'Thousands of drugs are used in medical practice,' and asks, 'Is it wise to dump so many into the human body when they are not included in the natural composition of the body?' He also said, '... Chemicals are life potencies; their atoms have attractions and repulsions, and to endeavour to introduce haphazard inorganic metals into an organic machine, is like feeding a baby with steel tacks to make it strong.'

Another point made by Ghadiali in this respect, is that deviation in the body above or below its normal percentage is a prime cause of illness, but doctors often unwittingly increase the imbalance, or reverse it to the opposite side, with their remedies: hence the many drug-induced illnesses.

Unreliable Drugs

Drugs can be unreliable, since people react

variously to different drugs. Witness the many people allergic to penicillin and allied drugs. In contrast, Chromotherapy leaves no harmful residues which the body has to work hard to eliminate. Chromotherapy does not treat symptoms, it goes to the root of the imbalance. Many of the illnesses to which man is heir have their root in the auric body and this can be seriously damaged by strong drugs. Chromotherapy uses the type of remedy which most closely matches the constituents of the auric bodies. It is the premise of Chromotherapy that by giving colour ray treatment instead of drugs, a constructive result can be obtained without any accompanying destructive effect.

In this respect it is interesting to note that for some reason the medical profession use the vibratory light spectrum just below and just above the visible light band, but are slow in acknowledging the healing properties of the visible light spectrum. Actually, of course, both infra-red and ultra-violet rays cause tissue damage if used to any sizeable extent, while the most which can occur by the use of an incorrect colour from the visible light spectrum, or if too long an exposure is given, is a temporary accentuation of a functional disorder.

In fact where both lay and medical therapists have used colour therapy they have been well pleased with the results.

CHAPTER TWO

THE AURA, CHAKRAS, AND SUBTLE BODIES

In the introduction, the electro-magnetic field which surrounds everything and which is known as the aura, was mentioned in relation to healing and diagnosis.

While the existence of the aura had always been known to occultists and clairvoyants, it was not until Dr W.J. Kilner of St Thomas's Hospital, London, accepted that it existed and began to experiment to make it visible to the human eye, that the ordinary person could see it. He developed the 'dicyanin screen', a lens painted with a coal-tar dye. This has a remarkable effect upon vision and enables the eye to perceive the ultra-violet range.

Medicine was in an exciting and progressive period at the time when young Dr Kilner joined the staff of St Thomas's Hospital. Contemporary researchers were Professor W.K. von Rontgen, discoverer of the x-ray, Dr Braid, whose work on the use of hypnosis is well known, and a German scientist, Carl von Reichenbach, who was publishing his findings on what he called 'odic force', a luminous emanation surrounding the body. At the same time – in the U.S.A. – Dr

Edwin Babbitt was engaged on his monumental work *The Principles of Light and Colour*. Great forces were advancing the scope of healing into fields hitherto forgotten, except by the few who inherited the wisdom of a vanished epoch.

Seeing the Aura

When Dr Kilner published his book, *The Human Atmosphere*, it was not well-received by orthodoxy, he was laughed at and discredited. However, he did not give up his experiments with the dicyanin screen and continued until the First World War cut off his supply of dicyanin, which was produced in Germany. Using the Kilner screen and working within the ultra-violet range, the aura can be seen as an inner band outlining the body, while a second band of almost vaporous light extends away from the body.

Through use of the Kilner screen the eyes become sensitized and so the aura may be seen as a grey-blue emanation. The most orthodox doctor could avail himself of this screen and so examine the condition of his patient, for the aura shows a dark or discoloured mark over the affected area.

Esoteric science gives a man a sevenfold nature of subtle bodies and the aura is the expression of that nature. The teaching is that man has not only got a physical body, but that he has, so to speak, a foot on other planes of being beyond the physical. Few will dispute that man has an intellectual and an emotional nature and so can, in common with his fellow human beings, operate on these planes as well as through his physical body.

The seven aspects of man are not separate states distinct from one another, but are currents of thought and feeling within the whole ocean of consciousness, and often overlap. Man then is a more complex creature than orthodox science allows or knows, for potentially he has these seven aspects which make up his complete being, but of course many people at present experience very little development on the higher vehicles.

The sevenfold division of man's nature is usually classified in the following levels of consciousness:

1. Physical Etheric Plane
2. Astral Plane
3. Lower Mental Plane
4. Higher Mental Plane
5. Spiritual Causal Plane
6. Intuitional Plane
7. Divine or Absolute Plane

To the skilled clairvoyant, or one who uses the Kilner screen, the aura will reveal a man's character, his emotional and mental nature, his state of health and his spiritual development.

Man being – as the Ancient Wisdom has always contended – a septenary being, the auric emanation consists of seven distinct units or waves of light, encircling the subject in an oval-shaped conformation. The extent and strength of the aura varies considerably from person to person, depending on his state of health, mental and emotional state, and his evolutionary status.

Man's Seven Subtle Bodies

The *first* aura is the one emanating from the physical etheric body and it is this cloud-shaped formation that most people see first when they practise seeing the aura. Its base is the centre of the spine. The etheric body, the vital counterpart of the physical, is important as it draws in the prana or life energy from the atmosphere and distributes it through the system.

In a healthy body the first aura radiates outwards in straight regular lines from the body's centre. In disease these lines are seen to droop, rather like bent lightning conductors.

The *second* aura emanates from the astral, or the emotional centre in the spleen, and encircles the astral body, extending about twelve to eighteen inches from the body. Every change of thought or emotion causes a change in this aura. It vibrates and changes continually. In harmony, it should be bright and luminous, showing emotional balance.

The *third* aura is the expression of man's intellectual make-up and its strength depends upon the development of his faculties, which in turn partly depends upon the education he has enjoyed. It is oval, emitting a radiant pale yellow colour as it develops. In the intelligent, well-balanced person, the aura is bright and shiny, but where the mind is depraved there are dark spots which dull its brightness.

The *fourth* aura is the emanation of man's higher mind or soul principle. Its colour tone is green. Here we have the realm of imagination, inspiration and intuition, of creativity in art and literature.

The *fifth* aura interpenetrates the foregoing auras. This aura manifests the essence of spirit in man. Occult science teaches us that conditions in the lower forms of consciousness are the result of forces within the spiritual body. It is the receiving station for all the doings of the lower aspects and records the impressions received by them. The fifth aura is most important, for it is the point of union between the cosmos and the individual. There exists a delicate band between the individual life and the ocean of consciousness shared by all.

The *sixth* and *seventh* auras are higher ones belonging rather to cosmic aspects than to individuals in particular. The average man has just not developed that high, and these auras would only be seen around the bodies of initiates and masters.

Chakras (Power Centres)

So we all have seven subtle bodies or levels of consciousness, ranging from the grossest, the physical, to the most spiritual or finest. These seven bodies all interpenetrate and are joined to the physical at the seven power centres or *chakras* in the spine. Through these centres and the rays which they attract we are in touch with, and affected by, all the seven planes of consciousness.

Each chakra attracts to itself a predominant colour ray which is necessary to the harmony of the whole individual.

A condition of disharmony implies that either too much or too little of a particular colour vibration is present. This may occur through some agency affecting us from outside, such as an accident or epidemic, or inwardly through the mind entertaining too many negative thoughts and so changing the vibrations in this way.

A small boy, upon being asked how he would describe God, said simply, 'I think of Him as Light.' Looked at from the angle of colour and its place in our lives, this is a very apt description, for all life is energy vibrating at a different rate. Each vibration has a corresponding colour and all colour rays emanate from the central source, the *Great White Light* or *Logos*, as we are instructed by the Ancient Teachings. In fact, as with everything else in life, there is an outer form to be perceived by our senses and an inner or hidden meaning to be discovered. So we come to discuss the chakras, through which the primal energy in the shape of white light, is drawn into the body through the power centres. Each chakra absorbs a special current of vital energy through its particular colour ray from the physical environment and from higher levels of consciousness.

In the completely healthy body the energy flows in harmoniously, and is absorbed through the chakras. The opposite occurs, however, where there is a blockage of one kind or another in one of the bodies.

If the cosmic energy stopped at the fourth level, say, then there would be some distortion in the way of thinking and this distortion would be transmitted to the astral and the physical/etheric bodies and so be experienced as some form of illness or dis-harmony in the physical body. The higher bodies affect the lower, but not vice versa.

*The Seven
Primary Rays*

*Centres which predominantly attract
these Rays*

1.	Red	The lowest centre in the base of the spine.
2.	Orange	In the small of the back, to the left-hand side of the spine. (Splenic centre.)
3.	Yellow	Middle of the back over the kidneys. (Solar plexus centre.)
4.	Green	Between the shoulder blades in line with the heart.
5.	Blue	At the base of the skull. (Throat centre.)
6.	Indigo	In the forehead, the pineal gland. (Brow centre.)
7.	Violet	In the dome of the head. (Pituitary centre.)

There are seven main chakras, each under a particular colour. These are seen clairvoyantly as continually moving great wheel-like vortices situated in the etheric body — the pattern on which the physical is built. These chakras or vortices link with the spine at definite intervals.

Light is a force stimulating to growth; every

living thing depends upon it to build and maintain its form. Light therefore, whose source is solar energy, is one of the greatest healing forces. In the human being energy is drawn in through the chakras and distributed over the whole body. The chakras draw in their own specialized colours, as listed above, so that the two lowest centres, the *red* and *orange*, draw in energy from the sunlight and this energy is directed through the body.

The *red and the orange chakras* govern the physical and etheric level in man and supply the vital energies needed by these bodies, although it should be mentioned that the activity of the chakras is not localized but interpenetrative. The *yellow chakra* governs the lower mental level, but also has to do with emotional influences. The *green chakra*, called the heart centre, governs the higher mind but also influences the higher emotions such as sympathy, kindness, understanding and compassion. The *blue or throat chakra* is the centre of religious and spiritual instincts. The *blue*, *red* and *yellow chakras* need to work in harmony for there to be genuine health of mind and body.

The *indigo* and *violet chakras* are both transcendental and rule the higher aspirations of the soul. These can express clairvoyance, spiritual intuition, or healing.

Colour healing can thus restore the balance where disease has caused a *blocking* or slowing down of the energy intake through the chakras or its circulation.

Diagnosis is made by clairvoyance, or by the use of aids to make the aura visible to those without psychic vision. The discoloured area showing disease can be treated by rays to clear the blockages. Colour breathing can also be advocated to hasten recovery or simply to maintain good health. Clairvoyant vision shows that where the aura is ragged or droopy and colour breathing is practised, there is an immediate revival of the frayed aura with the new intake of vitality.

Just as each major colour has seven intrinsic elements in its composition, so – according to the following table – in each colour one of the seven elements predominates. For instance, in number one a physical element predominates, this is the lowest centre at the base of the spine. In number five a specific healing element predominates, this is the throat centre and its colour is *blue*.

Base centre	1.	A physical element.
Splenic centre	2.	A vitality element.
Solar plexus centre	3.	A psychological element.
Heart centre	4.	A harmonizing element.
Throat centre	5.	A specific healing element.
Brow centre	6.	An element of inspiration and intuition.
Pituitary centre	7.	A spiritual element.

A Spiritual Force

Colour healing is not only a physical but a spiritual force, and so forms a link between our physical bodies and the finer forces or vibrations of higher levels of consciousness and spiritual growth. The use is not confined to spiritual or unorthodox healers, it is also used by orthodox practitioners, although perhaps the latter tend to use the more dangerous – because more powerful – infra-red and ultra-violet rays. However, it is possible that colour healing could also be the link or bridge between the orthodox and unorthodox disciplines, so that in the end the old orthodox idea of treating the physical body alone may die the death and new ideas, taking into account the wholeness of man and his entire *force field*, may benefit humanity mightily. It has many advantages over other methods of healing, being harmless and able to reach the subtle bodies, where all disease starts. Furthermore it makes possible early diagnosis through auric examination long before the disease manifests in the physical body, and it cannot cause side effects.

CHAPTER THREE

THE SEVEN MAJOR RAYS

As explained in the previous chapter, cosmic energy in the shape of light rays is drawn into the body through the chakras or power centres, distributed along the spine, and so flows through the body vitalizing it. Where there are blockages for whatever reason, this impoverishes the body and disease sets in.

The theory on which colour healing is based is that everyone is individual in their requirements of specific colours and that health of mind and body is based upon the body obtaining a balanced flow according to their requirements. That is, sufficient to enable the body to rebuild, restore and revitalize every organ in order to maintain its health and freedom from disease.

Just as man has seven bodies or levels of consciousness, so there are seven chakras and seven major rays.

The Red Cosmic Ray

This is the ray which supplies our physical bodies with energy and vitality. It is drawn in through the *base chakra* at the root of the spine and correlates with the *coccygeal* or *gonad centre*. The physical vitality of the body depends upon the correct and sufficient intake of the *red* ray, particularly so far as the creative, procreative and restorative functions are concerned.

Treatment with the *red* ray stimulates this centre. It promotes heat and body temperature, stimulates the circulation of the blood and gets the adrenalin going. It disperses feelings of tiredness and inertia, as well as chronic chills or colds; its action is always expansive. Diet to help the action of *red* rays should include beet, radishes, black cherries, damsons, plums, spinach, cresses and currants – in fact any vegetables and fruits containing iron. Healers also often suggest that the patient drink several tumblerfuls of *red* ray-charged water. This is water that has absorbed the *red* rays from the sun being filtered through a red screen. The effect of the *red* ray, psychologically and on the nervous system, is always uplifting, giving more confidence, initiative, overcoming depression and inertia, stimulating will-power and courage.

The use of the *red* ray could be indicated in cases of anaemia, paralysis, poor circulation, and disorders of the blood where the vitality is depleted or the mental state is one of depression, fear or worry.

The Orange Cosmic Ray
The *orange* ray controls the *second chakra*, the *splenic centre*, and it assists in the assimilative, distributory and circulatory processes of the body. It has a powerful tonic effect; frees the bodily and mental functions, gives both physical

energy and mental stimulation. It has often been called *the wisdom ray*. Lying as it does midway between the physical *red* ray, and the mental *yellow* ray, it has an action on both the physical vitality and the intellect. Diet to help the action of the *orange* rays includes most orange-skinned vegetables and fruits, oranges, tangerines, apricots, mangoes, peaches, cantaloup melons, carrots and swedes, also a glass or two of orange-charged water.

Both the *orange* and *red* rays are powerful and treatment should never be indiscriminately used. Each patient is unique and must be treated as such.

Psychologically, the *orange* ray is wonderful for removing repressions and inhibitions, it helps to broaden the mind and to open it to new ideas, where there is mental regardation it is a great help in raising the mental level. As it broadens the mind, it brings more understanding and tolerance. Like the *red* ray it also supplies courage and the power to cope with life.

As the *orange* ray is absorbed through the *splenic centre*, so it can be used for the treatment of disorders and infections of the spleen, also for kidney diseases. Bronchitis and other chest troubles can be treated with the *orange* ray. Gallstones respond to treatment by the *orange* ray, as does paralysis of any emotional origin.

The Yellow Cosmic Ray
Next to white, this is the ray giving out the maximum light, it is absorbed through the *third*

chakra, or the solar plexus, which is really a very important centre for the whole nervous system and it controls the digestive processes as well. Its action is eliminative on the liver and intestines so that it is a purifier for the whole system, but particularly for the skin, where it has powerful healing properties. It is a *mental ray*, and stimulates the intellectual faculties. Diet to help the action of the *yellow* ray consists basically of yellow skinned vegetables and fruit such as lemons, bananas, grapefruit, pineapples and sweetcorn. Again, many healers charge water in sunlight through a yellow filter and prescribe it for their patients.

Psychologically, the *yellow* ray stimulates the logical mind and the reasoning powers. It also aids self-control through inspiring the higher faculties. We are stimulated and our spirits raised by merely looking at yellow and orange, for these colours resemble most closely the lovely golden sunshine which our bodies crave. So yellow is a colour which brings a harmonious attitude to life, providing balance and optimism.

The use of the yellow ray could be indicated in cases of nervous exhaustion, where there are skin troubles, indigestion and the related complaints of constipation, liver trouble, diabetes.

The Green Cosmic Ray

Green is the colour of nature, of balance, peace and harmony. When we who live in the towns seek refreshment and contentment, we drive out into the country, even if this can only be for a few hours on Sundays! Instinctively we know that the green of the countryside will be restorative and soothing. It is the *midway* mark in the colour spectrum between the heat end of the spectrum and the electric end.

This is the *ray* which is absorbed by the *heart chakra* and controls the *cardiac centre*. *Green* is a mixture of blue and yellow, and strongly influences the heart and blood-pressure. In fact chlorophyll, which is produced by plants, can now be chemically synthesized, and is produced and marketed for sustaining the heart action. It also has a wonderful soothing effect upon the nerves and probably it is its lack in some of the built-up areas and concrete jungles designed by modern architects that accounts for the rising waves of crime and delinquency. Diet to help the action of the *green* ray is the use of all green vegetables and fruits that are neither acidulous nor alkaline in reaction.

Psychologically the *green* ray brings a feeling of renewal, of new life, freshness and brightness, rather like the coming of spring. This is the ray which governs not only the *physical* heart, but also emotional problems and repressions which bring on *heart attacks*; these are often due to a fear of giving, a fear of involvement or of being hurt; if these emotional and psychological problems continue over a long period they can all too easily end up in high blood-pressure and heart attacks.

Therefore, the *green* ray, experienced by getting away from it all into the country or at least into your garden, is a wonderful 'builder-upper' and restorer for the heart, and also for blood-pressure and ulcers. It can also be used for alleviating headaches and 'flu. As cancer is an imbalance of the cells, so *green*, the harmonizer and balancer, can be used to neutralize the extreme disharmony of malignant cells, restore harmony to the nervous system and tune up the whole body.

The Blue Cosmic Ray
Just as the *red* ray is an expander and stimulator, so the *blue* ray is the opposite, for it is the contractor and restrictor, so far as the previous group of *red/orange/yellow* rays are concerned. It is the 'steadier-upper' and slows things down so that it can combat infectious diseases where there is a rise in temperature. Its great property is that of an antiseptic, its light is cooling and astringent. *Blue* is the colour of the throat centre – the centre which controls man's greatest power of self-expression, speech. Diet to help the action of the *blue* ray consists of all blue fruits and vegetables such as grapes, blackberries, which are often a deep blue, blue plums, bilberries, and the taking of a glass or so of blue-charged water every day.

Psychologically, the *blue* ray can bring quiet and peace of mind, particularly where there has been an over-excited state, such as one bordering on hysteria. It can in fact be so relaxing that the common saying, 'I feel blue', would imply too much blue and the need for a little 'zip up and go' *red* or *orange*.

The *blue* ray can be used to alleviate many

diverse ailments such as throat troubles of all kinds, fevers and children's ailments, such as measles and mumps, many inflammations, spasms, stings, itchings and headaches. It is also useful for shock, insomnia and periodic pains.

The Indigo Cosmic Ray

The *indigo* ray is drawn in and circulated by the chakra behind the brow, often called *the third eye*. It is said to control the *pineal gland*, and is a wonderful purifier of the blood stream. Like the *orange ray*, it helps to broaden the mind and free it of fears and inhibitions. *Indigo* is a combination of *deep blue* and a small amount of steadying *red*.

The *pineal gland* has to do with the nervous, mental and psychic potential of a man, so that the organs of sight and hearing are under the influence of the *indigo* ray. It is probably for this reason that the *indigo* ray is a powerful anaesthetic – this is a very safe way of gaining anaesthesia for consciousness is maintained, but there is complete insensitivity to pain. Diet to help the action of the *indigo* ray can include the foods listed under the *blue* ray and those which will be given for the *violet* ray too.

Psychologically, it clears and cleans the psychic currents of the body. It even has a powerful effect on serious mental complaints such as obsession and other forms of psychosis. The *indigo* ray is purifying and stabilizing where fears and repressions have produced a serious mental complaint.

In treatment the *indigo* ray can be used to treat

any diseases of the eyes, ears and nose, also diseases of the lungs, asthma and dyspepsia. Deafness can sometimes be the result of a refusal to hear the voice of conscience or enlightenment, or merely the words of those close to the patient. Instead there is an in-turning of attention. Naturally, this is not always so, but in any case the *indigo* ray can be of great help in any ear, nose, or throat problem.

The Violet Cosmic Ray

This is the highest vibration of all the cosmic energy rays. It controls the *crown chakra* in the head, and is linked with the *pituitary gland*, which is a centre of intuitive and spiritual understanding. The *violet* ray acts in a most soothing and tranquillizing manner upon frayed nervous systems, of which there are plenty today. However, its usefulness in terms of response is mainly for those who are nervous and highly-strung by nature. Artists, actors and musicians; these often suffer from personality disorders and it is the violet ray which can restore them to peace and calm.

Diet to be used together with charged waters, are such foods as recommended for the *indigo* ray, and aubergines, purple grapes, blackberries, purple broccoli, beetroot.

Psychologically, this is the *ray de luxe*, which has a wonderful healing effect on all forms of neurosis and neurotic manifestations. It can be used to assist the development of the spiritual, intuitive faculty. Before beginning meditation or concentration exercises, the colour could be visualized or else a small cloth of that colour could be placed on a table in front of you as an aid to stimulating the psychic and spiritual faculties.

In treatment *violet* can be used for all mental and nervous disease, also for rheumatism, concussion, tumours, cerebro-spinal meningitis, kidney and bladder diseases.

The *ancient wisdom* teaches that colour names and the numbers of each *chakra* and ray are symbols for great forces which emanate from the Supreme power behind all manifestation. Each of the seven rays stands for one of the great evolutionary periods through which humanity has to pass. Everything in existence is dependent upon these great cosmic radiations, not only this earth, but all the other planes of manifestation, the etheric, astral, mental and spiritual planes which make up the universe, all are dependent on this same cosmic power of Light.

The *seven rays* represent stages in evolutionary progress. The first three rays, the *red, orange* and *yellow*, have already been past, humanity is now in the evolutionary period of the *green ray*, the mid-point and the lowest point of immersion in matter. Ahead the outlook is brighter, a period of progress awaits humanity, with an advance into the higher, more harmonious *blue ray* and so to the finer conditions of the *indigo* and *violet rays*.

As these rays and their numbers are symbols of great *Forces* with which we are surrounded every day of our lives, so each one of us has command of particular gifts which are part of our own potential for development in terms of material or creative success, and this we will see in a later chapter devoted to music, colour and number in our lives.

Dr Edwin D. Babbit in his classic work *The Principles of Light and Colour* (published in 1878), tells us how, after many years of research into colour therapy, he developed the ability with his inner vision to see colours swirling around him in a great ocean of flashing light, and describes the experiences as being beyond belief in glory. Everything became a mass of luminous, swirling radiations flowing into, through, and from, everything. He concluded that there was a basically spiritual force from which *all* healing must come of whatever nature. It is simply the channels we use to effect the healing that differ.

CHAPTER FOUR

DIAGNOSIS AND TREATMENT

When we think about healing we usually consider only the physical body of flesh and muscle that we can see, but it is well to remember that the Ancient Wisdom teaches that this body consists of two parts, one visible and the other invisible or 'subtle'. This latter is the vital body or 'etheric double'. Both are composed of physical matter and both are cast off at death. The etheric body is the source of all physical vitality and the absorber and transmitter of energy through the system. This double is an exact replica of the visible body, its organs corresponding exactly with the phsyical organism, hence disease begins first in the etheric body, or in one of the higher bodies, before it attacks the physical; there can, therefore, be an early diagnosis of the impending disease.

Two Nervous Systems

Operations of the physical organism depends upon the efficient functioning of the nervous systems, of which there are two. The Involuntary System, not under the control of the will, operates all the automatic functions of the body, such as heart beating and breathing, without our having to worry about them; in fact if we did we would probably stop their functioning.

The other nervous system is Voluntary and is centred on the brain, spinal cord and solar plexus. Through this system we think, feel and act. If these centres are defective in any way, man's expression in the physical world is imperfect to the extent of the damage.

Colour rays affect the condition of both the etheric and physical cells. This etheric body is the connecting link between the physical senses and the higher forces, and in health the vital or etheric body energizes the physical body. To clairvoyant or trained vision, the aura of the etheric body is visible as a luminous outline of a pale golden colour radiating outwards in every direction. These radiations, when strong and healthy, can get rid of germs and infections through their strength and vitality, but in ill health the etheric strength is depleted, unable to absorb the correct amount of energy, and the radiations – lacking vital force – appear to the clairvoyant as drooping lines.

Colour healing aims to build up the etheric body through applying the correct colour vibrations to the *chakras*, which then become capable of vitalizing the physical body.

Methods of Diagnosis

There are three main methods of diagnosis, by psychic perception, the use of the Kilner screen – whereby the conditions on the astral and etheric levels can be ascertained – and by radiesthesia, or the use of E.S.P. functioning through the pendulum.

I am told that practitioners can map the outline of the aura by using certain designs of the pendulum. To the radiesthetist each colour has its own particular vibration and this they can pick up by observing the swing of the pendulum. Allied to this is the diagnostic and treatment instrument; attunement is made through a sample spot of blood, a hair snippet or even a signature. An expert can make a complete health diagnosis and treat the patient.

The trained psychic is aware of the different levels of consciousness through which man works, his sevenfold potential contained within the one, all with their different radiations making up the aura or the ovoid electro-magnetic field with which we are all surrounded. Here is the outward expression of the man, his physical, emotional, lower and higher, mental and spiritual potentials. To the psychic, the dullness or patchiness of colour will be observable and treatment can be given at the required level. Some psychics are so gifted that they do not even require the presence of the patient, but can diagnose at a distance provided they have an article belonging to the person in their hands.

So far as the third method of diagnosis is concerned, by means of radiesthesia and the radionic instrument, this will be very similar to the psychic investigation and naturally will vary according to the training and experience of the practitioner.

The Kilner Screen

Finally we come to the method using the Kilner screen, pioneered by Dr Kilner. He was convinced that it could be a much more effective way of diagnosis as ill health would show up in the aura before the physical symptoms appeared.

The Kilner screen is composed of two pieces of glass between which has been poured a solution of dicyanin, a dye of indigo-violet colour, which considerably sharpens the vision of the observer. Ideally a special diagnosing cabinet would be built where that patient can be seated, clad only in a black silk robe to facilitate vision. The condition of the lower auras can then be seen. If a special cabinet is not possible, then the diagnostician should seat the patient in a darkened room. After a while the emanations from the etheric body will become visible.

It should be mentioned that in emergency it is often necessary to diagnose through symptoms, the person's general demeanour, and expressed habits. Remember that there are two principal colours, the heating *red/orange* and the cooling *blue/violet*, green representing the mid-point, the balance or harmonizer.

Broadly the aim of the healer is to find out which of these opposing colours is wanting in the patient and how to cure the complaint. For instance, if the person is inclined to be depressed, is slow in reaction, has no energy or appetite, then he requires the *red/orange* colours rays. If he is impatient, choleric, overactive or has a raised temperature, he requires the *blue/violet* rays to cool him.

Locating the Diseased Organ

There are two main types of healing; contact and absent. In both cases the aim of healing is to restore the vitality to the etheric vehicle through the projection of colour rays; these are then absorbed by the power centres interpenetrating the spine. The decision as to which centre the ray should be directed to, will depend upon the position of the diseased organ.

Another method open to those with sensitive finger tips or hands – if psychic vision is not developed – is to pass the right hand over the body until the vibration of the fingers, or in some people the tingling of the palm and a heat sensation, show that the seat of the trouble has been located. This is somewhat similar to the use of the pendulum for diagnosis and either the hand or the pendulum could be used to pick out the colour ray to be used. Naturally a broad sample card of colours well depicted would have to be used for the latter method.

Treatment can be either diffused over the body or concentrated. Continuity of treatment is important and most healers seem to agree that treatment should last for about twenty-five to thirty minutes. Overall treatment consists in focusing the lamps, or in some cases the hands are used to direct the colour – through thought-power – over the whole body, but especially over the back. The patient either lies or sits in a relaxed position, with the upper half of the body uncovered. This is a wonderful tonic for revitalizing and toning up the body.

Coloured Filters

In concentrated treatment the colour lamp with the appropriate filter for the particular disharmony is focused on the affected area only. This treatment usually lasts about fifteen minutes and can be followed by the general overall one. Most healers use a lamp or projector into which different coloured filters can be inserted. A more elaborate electrical colour treatment apparatus is an Electro Thermolume cabinet. The patient sits in the cabinet and is bathed in colour from colour screens fixed at the front of the cabinet.

Another often used and effective method is through the use of colour solarized water. Dr Babbitt suggests that not only water can be charged, but also milk, sugar and pulverized gum arabic, as these substances are fairly neutral and so can be used to take any colour charge required. The method is either to place the water in a jar or a glass of the required colour and leave it out in sunlight for an hour or two, or to place coloured paper over the glass or jar, again of course of the required colour. The patient then drinks the solarized water.

Colour Breathing

Another method is colour breathing. Sit by an open window, relax and expel all the air from the lungs. Then breathe in the required colour visualized in your mind. Breathe in to a certain count, hold to a certain count, and exhale to the same count. It is hard to advise for everyone, so each should find whatever count it is which suits, and perhaps increase it as the vitality builds up – for example, starting with breathing in to a count of four, holding for a count of four, exhaling for a count of four.

Colour breathing is best done before or after breakfast or the evening meal – not last thing at night. One should visualize the first three *rays* as flowing up from the earth towards the solar plexus. The last three, *blue, indigo* and *violet* should be breathed in downwards from the air. The *green* ray can be visualized as flowing into the system horizontally.

Some colour therapists do not use any apparatus at all, but use their sensitive hands and direct them to the centre of trouble, visualizing the colour ray to be given. The right hand being the positive hand, is placed over the *solar plexus*, while the left hand is held over the *chakra* nearest to the seat of the trouble. This great nerve centre has been mentioned more than once before, because of its influence upon health. When the right or positive hand is placed on the solar plexus and the mind is visualizing and directing the correct healing ray, this enables the ray to flow through the nervous system. The healer's left hand completes the circuit.

After about five minutes the left hand can be withdrawn and later returned at the end of the treatment, which lasts as long as the healer feels necessary. When the left hand is returned a sweeping motion can be executed to withdraw any negative vibrations. Every healer will tell you to remember that the hands must be warm and that the treatment should finish with a short direction of colour to the spine.

A shorter version of the above is the *colour pass*, in which the hands alone are used to transmit colour to the patient. Again a necessary affirmation is made as to intent regarding the patient, such as, 'I will relieve Mrs X of her persistent headaches and will transmit the blue ray to restore harmony.' The healer – after concentrating on his intention and holding in mind the colour ray for transmission – makes a broad, circular sweep up over the patient's head, brings his hands together and sweeps them down in an outward movement from the patient's body, so throwing off the patient's negative vibrations.

Most healers advocate certain foods should be included in the patient's diet according to the type of colour ray needed; this was dealt with in an earlier chapter. They may of course also advise colour breathing and the drinking of a magnetized water.

Absent Healing Therapy

It seems pretty certain that much ill health is the result of wrong thinking. Habitual wrong thinking is impressed upon the subconscious mind, which is a creative faculty and can bring to pass those things which we constantly visualize and press upon it. Healing then can basically be thought of as a change of mental attitude.

We have to remember that long before man

began to develop his intellect and his conscious mind, his subconscious existed, forming as it does part of the universal *unconscious* common to everything that exists rooted in the dark past of the ages, and the individual unconscious is part of the whole.

In absent healing the therapist usually asks the patient to link with him at a specified time every day. He then has to identify closely with the patient on a mental level so that in this way he is able to influence the patient's unconscious and impress upon it thoughts of health and healing. At the same time he directs the right colour ray.

The patient is also asked to relax and be receptive. On the other hand the healer needs a positive direction to his energy, for he has to get through the patient's objective conscious mind and reach his subjective and unconscious side in order to make the healing effective. Both patient and healer are partners in a joint project and should be attuned to one another. The healer usually likes to have some article which serves as a link with the patient. As in contact healing, a positive affirmation is made and after the patient's name and problem is clearly set in the healer's mind this is proceeded with; however, the main essential is that the healer should either be a natural *visualizer*, able to see colour and hold it in his mind long enough to direct it, or he should have so trained his mind through concentration that he has become so.

Another method of absent healing is that of meditating about the patient in a positive sense, that is, seeing him as restored to health and happiness.

Every therapist is very well aware of the power of thought, so they always impress upon their patients the importance of eliminating all negative fearful thinking. Thoughts should be optimistic and the patient is recommended to visualize himself in happy conditions and in good health.

It seems pretty clear that whether the treatment be personal or by absent healing, the colour healer parts company in a very basic way with the orthodox practitioner in the latter's purely physical approach to disease. Like the radionic's expert, the colour therapist bases his diagnosis and treatment on the actual existence of various invisible – to the physical eye – bodies, particularly the etheric, emotional and mental. Both believe that any blocking or over-stimulation (at any level), of the energies which are taken in and circulated through the *chakras* causes disease.

For healing to be effective, the therapist must have the capacity to diagnose correctly and visualize clearly, so directing colour correctly to the healing of the patient, for energy follows thought. This requires not only the ability and the desire to heal, but also discipline and training on the part of the therapist.

CHAPTER FIVE

COLOURS FOR COMMON DISEASES

Diagnosis, by various methods, is directed at the etheric body and its seven major force centres. The condition and activity of these centres must first of all be assessed, for it is the force fields or the invisible bodies of man, and in particular the etheric, which form the framework or mesh on which the physical vehicle is built, and these determine the vitality activity and health of that body.

The therapist is well aware that correct breathing and adequate fresh air is necessary for health, and he will perhaps suggest exercises of colour breathing to supply the lacks he has diagnosed. He will also remind his patient of the value of sunlight, sea air and the countryside as being helpful to the building up of the vitality. Nor will he forget the part which vitamins play in supplying the necessary energy to the vital body. This becomes even more important as our food becomes more and more devitalized with additives and preservatives.

The Ancient Wisdom teachings identify seven major chakras along the spine and in the head. These are wheels of rotating subtle matter and represent energy centres. The organs of the body have affinity with each of these. The *red chakra* at the base of the spine controls the functioning of the *creative and reproductive system*. This is the focus for the treatment of these problems.

The *orange chakra* is centred on the *spleen*, and influences the process of digestion and assimilation. Treatment involving these should be focused on this centre. The *yellow chakra* lies in the *solar plexus*, and treatment is centred on this chakra where there is disharmony present in relation to *adrenal glands, pancreas and liver*. The *green chakra* is the *heart*. Diseases of the *heart*, the *blood and circulatory system* are treated through focusing on it. The *blue chakra* relates to the *throat* and is found at the back of the neck. Diseases to do with the *throat, thyroid* and *parathyroid glands* are treated via this chakra.

Indigo is the *forehead chakra*; it is located between the eyebrows and correlates with the *pituitary gland*. This is the master controlling gland for the *entire endocrine system*. It has to balance the under- or over-activity of the other glands and so may become overworked. Diseases of the *brain, eyes, nose, ears* and *nervous system* are treated by focusing on this chakra.

The following suggestions for treatment are derived from authorities on colour such as S.G.J. Ousley, Gladys Myer and Roland Hunt.

Red Ray

This is the element of fire. Stimulating and exciting the nerves and blood, it releases adrenalin, activates the circulation of the blood and vitalizes the physical body. Being a powerful stimulant it must be used with caution. It should never be used alone, but followed by green or blue. Contra-indications are inflammatory conditions, and emotional disturbances.

Anaemia
Red colour breathing will be important as well as the drinking of red-charged water. Foods should include fruits and vegetables listed under the red ray. Ousley, in his book *Power of the Rays*, suggests that red light should be administered with a colour lamp first to the soles of the feet and then on the red chakra at the base of the spine at a distance of about six inches. He suggests a progression of five minutes each on the soles of the feet, then the calves, knees, thighs and the base of the spine, finishing up with a few minutes of green or blue light.

Paralysis
In the first treatment or so, it is recommended by various therapists that yellow light should be used in order to help the patient reorientate his mental state, which is likely to be confused. Yellow should be directed to the patient either by thought or by lamps. Purple light should be administered to the base chakra for ten minutes. The same ray should be allowed to play lightly up the spine for about five minutes and then allowed to rest on the soles of the feet, on the knees and the legs for about ten minutes. However these times vary with each individual and should be sensed by the therapist or tested by the pendulum.

Orange Ray

It strengthens the lungs, pancreas and spleen, enlivens the emotions and creates a feeling of well-being. This is a stimulating, warming colour, an anti-spasmodic, and can – like the red ray – be used for lack of vitality, and muscle spasms or cramps. A general diffusion of light should be given over the whole body, then concentrated on the solar plexus and the base of the brain for ten to fifteen minutes.

Asthma

Again the orange ray is the one to use, although it is more imperative than usual that correct breathing is practised and the exercise of breathing in the orange ray should be done faithfully every day. Deep breathing, in which the lungs are properly cleared using the deep muscles of the chest and stomach, is most important. Also the mental attitude needs to be positive and optimistic. Treatment is the directing of the orange ray on to the chest and throat for ten minutes at a time. As improvement is shown, the *blue ray* directed to the throat for fifteen minutes will be found helpful. The drinking of orange charged water also helps the condition.

Bronchitis

This is not a condition which responds easily to treatment, particularly if the condition is a long-standing one. For treatment the orange light is focused on the stomach and abdomen for the usual ten to fifteen minutes, or longer according to the patient's need. Orange and lemon juice have proven helpful for this condition and should be taken regularly. Again colour breathing of the orange ray should be followed.

Faulty Elimination

This is a condition which may show itself in vertical ridging of the finger and toe nails, but sometimes exists unsuspected by the patient because there is no outward sign of ill health. However it does respond rapidly to the administration of the orange ray and the drinking of orange-charged water taken twice daily.

Epilepsy

This is not an easy condition to cure once the disease has become established. However, treatment is by the blue ray to the head and the drinking of orange-charged water daily.

Yellow Ray

Activates the motor nerves and generates energy in the muscles, stimulates the flow of bile, is good for the skin, psychologically it can get rid of depression. This is a positive vibration and acts on the nervous system, influencing the mental attitude and the bodily vitality. The solar plexus centre is the most critical of all for the vitalization of the whole body, acting as it does as an assimilator and distributor of energies to the other chakras.

Dyspepsia
This condition may be caused by either too much red or too much blue in the system. Distinction may be made by the fact that those who draw in too much red are usually thin, while those who draw in too much blue are usually fat and lacking in vitality. Deep colour breathing of the yellow ray and the drinking of yellow-charged water should be practised during the day. The solar plexus should be exposed to yellow twice daily for thirty minutes. The antidote to an excess of red is the blue ray, as this reduces the irritation and restores health.

Diabetes
With this condition the blood becomes impoverished. The yellow light should be directed in the solar plexus centre for fifteen minutes twice daily and the yellow-charged water also taken twice daily. This reduces the formation of fat in the cells and allows the condition of the blood to return to normal. Treatment will be lengthy.

Flatulence
Treatment for this condition is basically simply the drinking of yellow-charged water slowly between meals.

Constipation
The yellow light should be directed to the stomach and abdomen for twenty minutes night and morning. Colour breathing of the yellow ray

should be practised and small quantities of yellow-charged water taken between meals. Yellow is contra-indicated in acute inflammation, fever, over-excitement and heart palpitation. However, too much yellow can bring on diarrhoea, as it stimulates the flow of bile.

Green Ray

Ray of harmony and balance, it is nature's tonic and exercises a strong influence on the heart and on the blood supply. Green relieves tension, it stimulates the pituitary gland and builds muscle and tissue.

Heart Complaints: Blood-pressure

Most therapists are agreed that heart complaints originate in the emotional body and are often due to an excitable nervous system. Green light focused on the heart centre helps to harmonize and heal. Visualization of the colour emerald by the patient is of help too. For low blood-pressure the quality of light directed to the patient should be dark and treatment last for thirty minutes. In high blood-pressure, a pale green light should be used for the same length of time. Green-charged water should be taken and plenty of green vegetables included in the diet.

Headaches

Treatment of these should be by means of diffused light over the whole body. Response is usually rapid.

Blue Ray

This ray is cold and astringent in quality. It is a ray with antiseptic qualities. It controls the throat chakra and produces a calm, peaceful vibration. It is called for in any feverish or inflamed condition as it is the antidote to red. Contra-indicated for colds, paralysis, chronic rheumatism and hypertension.

Sore Throat

The blue light should be focused on the throat for fifteen minutes and the patient asked to gargle with blue-charged water every two hours.

Hoarseness

The blue-charged water should be taken in small doses and the throat given treatment by the blue light for half-an-hour. Blue ray breathing will help if done on rising.

Goitre

Treatment is directing the blue light to the throat for half-an-hour and gargling with the blue-charged water as frequently as possible until the condition improves.

Fevers

In all fevers the blue light should be focused on the centre of the inflammation.

Palpitation

Small doses of blue-charged water, alternating

with green-charged water has been found to improve the condition.

Bilious Attacks
Blue-charged water taken every hour acts most effectively.

Colic
One ounce of blue-charged water taken every hour is beneficial for this condition.

Jaundice
Treatment is by a diffusion of blue light over the whole body. Small doses of blue-charged water also prove beneficial.

Cuts and Burns
Application of the blue-charged water will help to take away the pain and assist healing. Use of the blue ray stops bleeding.

Rheumatism
Where the condition is acute the blue light can be used effectively. Where the condition is chronic, the orange ray is called for.

Indigo Ray
Is cooling, astringent and electric. It works on the parathyroid glands, but depresses the thyroid. It reduces bleeding and also affects the emotional and spiritual levels. One can get rid of obsessions with it. Its use is called for in diseases of the ear, eye and nose; it is also beneficial in the treatment

of certain nervous and mental disorders. Can also
be used in the treatment of lung complaints and
stomach troubles.

Deafness

It has been found that this condition is often due
to unhappiness and introversion in childhood –
the child learns to go inward and shut himself
away from others so that an effort to be more
outgoing once the complaint begins to improve
often helps a great deal.

The indigo light should be directed to the ear,
or ears, and colour breathing of the indigo ray
practised night and morning. At the same time
the ear or ears should be bathed with indigo-
charged water once a day.

Cataract

Therere are two stages of treatment. In the first,
indigo ray breathing should be practised and the
eyes bathed with indigo-charged water. Cloths
wrung out with the charged water should be laid
on the forehead.

In the second stage of treatment, the indigo
light is directed to the eyes and forehead for
thirty minutes daily.

Inflamed Eyes and Ears

Inflammation of the eye can sometimes be due to
digestive disturbances; in these cases both the
blue and indigo rays can be directed to the face
and the head.

Earache responds to treatment by indigo light

and indigo-charged water should be taken twice daily.

Pneumonia
This is an excellent and speedy remedy for pneumonia. Treatment by indigo ray lowers the temperature, and heals the lungs.

Mental Disorders
The indigo ray has been found to be effective in the treatment of mental disorders when the patient is violent and excitable. Where the patient is depressed and inert the orange rays give results.

Violet Ray
Depresses the motor nerves and the lymphatic and cardiac systems. It purifies the blood and stops the growth of tumour. It maintains the potassium balance in the body. These are used quite extensively in orthodox medicine, but it is a powerful and subtle vibration and acts on man's highest body so that its use is contra-indicated where the mind is retarded or undeveloped. It controls the pituitary body.

Nervous Ailments
The use of this ray is called for when the patient is under a great deal of stress and strain and is a highly-strung and creative person. The opposite colour yellow cheers and raises the spirits when depression sets in and can be used in these cases.

Colour breathing and the drinking of colour-charged water is also beneficial.

Insomnia
Treatment by violet ray can be most effective in combating insomnia, especially where the patient is highly-strung and sensitive. However, both the calm rays of the blue and the indigo light have been used effectively.

Mental Disorders
It may be found that the violet ray is more effective in treating excitable cases than the indigo ray mentioned earlier. The blue ray is also often found to have a calming and soothing effect on the brain and so is helpful in the treatment of mental disorders.

Eye Troubles
Treatment by the violet ray can often be as effective as the indigo and the same process of treatment is recommended.

Gem Therapy
Gem therapy, like colour therapy, homoeopathy and radionic practice, approaches healing from the same angle; that of treating the whole man with all his physical and subtle bodies which form the force field surrounding and vitalizing his physical vehicle.

In colour healing, sunlight or electric light and various other methods are used to heal the patient. In gem therapy the seven principal gems are the source from which healing proceeds.

Allied to the personal treatment given by gem therapy where the patient has to come to the healer, a new treatment has been developed called teletherapy. Discs are set with gems and rotated by a small electric motor. The gems' rays fall on the patient's photograph and this link acts as a receiver of the rays and a conductor to the patient of the healing qualities of the gems' rays. This has, of course, great similarity to the treament given by radionic practitioners, where the healer has a snippet of hair, blood spot, or a photograph of the patient and broadcasts the homoeopathic remedy in the potency required.

Dr A. Bhattacharyya has a practice in Naihati, India, where he treats patients daily using gem remedies and treatment is also given by the teletherapy devices for reaching absent patients.

There is some difference between the colours of the gems used and the colours of the major rays used in colour healing proper; however both treat the chakras. The following are as described by Dr Bhattacharyya.

Ruby   Astrologically corresponding to the sun – cosmic red ray.
            It is recommended for heart diseases, circulatory problems, anaemia, loss of vitality, eye diseases and various mental troubles.

Pearl   Astrologically corresponding to the moon – orange cosmic ray.
            It is used for diabetes, asthma, gallstones, diarrhoea, menopausal difficulties.

Coral   Astrologically corresponding to Mars –
               yellow cosmic ray.
               Liver diseases, impure blood, high blood-
               pressure, skin troubles, haemorrhoids,
               sexual diseases.

Emerald   Astrologically corresponding to Mercury –
               green cosmic ray.
               Weak digestion, colic, cancer, skin
               problems, hypertension, heart troubles and
               ulcers.

Topaz   Astrologically corresponding to Jupiter –
               blue cosmic ray.
               Effectively treats any throat troubles,
               asthma, laryngitis, childhood infectious
               diseases, insomnia and shock.

Diamond   Astrologically corresponds to Venus –
               indigo cosmic ray.
               It is used for treating eye problems,
               vaious forms of paralysis, enlarged spleen,
               epilepsy.

All these have other indications and only a few are given above. Two other gems are frequently used; the *onyx*, which carries the ultra-violet frequency and can be used for bacterial or virus infection, and the *cat's eye*, giving off the infra-red frequency used for skin diseases, headaches and indigestion.

CHAPTER SIX

HEALTH FROM NUMBERS AND MUSIC

It is only too obvious that good health is the basis for all the other happinesses which life can offer us, so in this chapter I would like to make various suggestions for maintaining good health.

Each number represents a certain part of the body. The day of the month on which you are born will give a clue to the physical condition, and assist you through knowing your health, strength, and weaknesses.

Number One
Corresponds to the head and lungs. With many ones in the name, there is often a tendency to an inferiority complex and illness can too often result due to the lack of opportunity to make use of original ideas. For the 'number one', exercises in deep breathing are beneficial, even essential to success. Remember in adding up to your birthdate, 'number ones' are not only those born on the first, but also those born on the twenty-eighth or any number which reduces to *one*, for example, $2 + 8 = 10 = 1$. Always reduce your birthdate to a single figure.

Number Two
Corresponds to the nervous system, brain and

solar plexus. The physical body is sensitive and impressionable. Very affected by noise, hard conditions and coarse assocations. The feelings are sensitive, the person easily hurt and this can lead to illness and poor health generally. Diet is very important to maintain good health. Periods of rest and relaxation in a harmonious environment are helpful.

Number Three
Corresponds to the throat, tongue, larynx and the organs of speech. Many Three people become ill due to emotional disturbances, the feeling of lack of popularity and a general worrying tendency about the self. It is advisable for number Threes to cultivate a less pessimistic attitude to life and to worry less about what others think of them.

Number Four
Corresponds to the stomach, the right arm and the upper right side of the body. Rich foods should be avoided as this causes high blood-pressure and overweight. One of the most enduring of numbers, but even their endurance can be worn down by long periods of hard work and worry. The Fours should avoid taking themselves and life too seriously, as this can lead to lack of energy and circulatory problems.

Number Five
Corresponds to the liver, gall bladder, the left arm and the upper left side of the body. With

many people born on a Five day, overactivity, restlessness, inner dissatisfaction and critical states of mind bring nervous tension, the bane of the Five; this upsets the whole physical co-ordination. Fives are subject to accidents and physical hurts entailing long periods of convalescence.

Number Six
Corresponds to the heart, blood and skin. With many Sixes, heart trouble is likely to be organic, not the sudden heart attacks so often found today, these belong more to Fours and Fives. Domestic problems, the affairs of children and lack of love tend to bring about chronic conditions with many Sixes. Sixes need good planning in their domestic affairs and attention to diet.

Number Seven
Corresponds to the spleen, white blood cells and the sympathetic nervous system. These are selective people generally, but they need to be so regarding diet, and also periods of relaxation are necessary and escape from too public a life. Repression of the emotions and feelings often give poor physical health. The lower left side of the body and the left leg are often affected.

Number Eight
Corresponds to the colon, eyes and bowels. Nervous indigestion, nervous headaches and ulcers result from an over-active and intense way

of living; ambition often drives the Eight too hard. Of all the numbers, the Eight has both the greatest endurance and the most ability to recover. Sport and relaxation keeps the body healthy.

Number Nine
Corresponds to the kidneys and generative organs, also diseases hard to diagnose, brought about by self-indulgence and wrong habits of living. Alcohol or drugs are taboo for the Nines. Good health depends upon not being too impressionable or living too much in the clouds. Their escapist tendency can often be their undoing.

Each number has its characteristic colour, according to its rate of vibration. Each of the numbers mark strength and weaknesses, so a little care will help you maintain good health.

Number	Corresponding colour
1	Red
2	Orange
3	Yellow
4	Green
5	Blue
6	Indigo
7	Purple/Violet
8	Opal
9	Carmine

It should be noted that number nine is all colour, for it contains within it all other colours.

Using the above colour key you can analyse your name and discover your key colour vibration.

The main meanings of the character in relation to the numbers are:

Vibration	Number	Meaning
Red	1	Love and will power.
Orange	2	Constructivity and joy.
Yellow	3	Intellectual power.
Green	4	Self-control.
Blue	5	Faith and aspiration.
Indigo	6	Integration.
Purple	7	Transmutation of desires.
Opal	8	Understanding of life.
Carmine	9	Compassion.

The relationship of the numbers to the letters are:

Numbers	Letters
1	AJS
2	BKT
3	CLU
4	DMV
5	ENW
6	FOX
7	GPY
8	HQZ
9	IR

If we take an example this will make the matter clearer. Take two names we all know well.

HAROLD JAMES WILSON
8 1 9 6 3 4   1 1 4 5 1   5 9 3 1 6 5

Here we have:

Numbers	Vibrations
5 ones	Red
no twos	Orange
2 threes	Yellow
2 fours	Green
3 fives	Blue
2 sixes	Indigo
no sevens	Purple/Violet
1 eight	Opal
2 nines	Carmine

There is a preponderance of the red vibration, a common one in leaders, giving Harold Wilson a very strong will. There are however certain *lacks*, namely on the orange vibration of constructivity and joy and on the purple or violet vibration of transmutation of desires. It follows that to balance his nature, Harold Wilson needs to wear in some part of his clothing a tie or handkerchief in orange or purple

He has the capacity for leadership through love rather than through force. He has faith and aspiration (three blue vibrations), a certain mystical quality, he has intellectual ability (the yellow vibration), and compassion (the carmine vibration), and self-control (green vibration).

If we take the second well known name, we have:

EDWARD GEORGE HEATH
5 4 5 1 9 4   7 5 6 9 7 5   8 5 1 2 8

Translated these become:

Numbers	Vibrations
2 ones	Red
1 two	Orange
no threes	Yellow
2 fours	Green
5 fives	Blue
1 six	Indigo
2 sevens	Violet
2 eights	Opal
2 nines	Carmine

In this case there is a predominance of the five (blue vibration), giving faith and aspiration, which is his predominating quality, rather than the will/leadership of Harold Wilson. The other colours he has in balance, giving him the love/will/leadership of the red ray, the self-control of the green ray, the transmutation of desires through the violet ray, an understanding of life of the opal vibration, and compassion of the carmine ray. He has only one lack, that of the yellow vibration, intellectual power. This does not mean that other colours cannot compensate for this lack, in fact he has better, he has a balance on the higher colours of opal and carmine, giving him an understanding of people and a great sympathy for them, to be transmuted into his sure faith that he can help to make it practical.

Edward Heath needs to wear a touch of yellow to compensate for his lack on the intellectual level, but he already has a predominance of the

Soul Mind colour of blue and so this is not a grave lack. Visualization of the colours lacking in the name can also help to rectify imbalances in the character, in this case, reasonableness and logical thought can be lifted to wisdom.

Negative Attributes

Naturally, all the colour attributes can be used negatively, the red ray can become resentment, conceit, lack of compassion. The orange ray used negatively can promote destructiveness and despair or flamboyant exhibitionism. The green ray used negatively, can become a perpetual sense of injustice and ingrained grievance, and produce attitudes of rigid fixation where more flexibility and less serious intensity would help. The blue ray can, too easily, degenerate into selfish ambition, faith can become faithlessness, trust degenerate into distrust and serenity into dullness, apathy and lack of spirit.

Negatively the indigo ray can lead people in the ways of intolerance, separativeness, with disintegration usurping the unity of integration. Obsessive illusions can poison the mind.

The violet/purple ray used negatively can portray snobbishness and overweening self-esteem, while the perversity of the purple ray is associated with arrogance, fanaticism and treachery. The opal ray used negatively produces vaunting ambition, love of power and position, a completely materialist philosophy which ignores the rights of others and strives for self-advancement, power and more power.

The carmine ray used negatively works for self alone, has little thought for humanity and the brotherhood of man. Greed, selfishness and love of material things is the perversion of this ray.

To help promote happiness and health it is a good thing to be mindful of your own basic physical constitution as shown by the day of birth and its addition to a single digit. Wear the colour of your birthday from time to time so as to be in harmony with your basic ray colour. It is also beneficial to wear the colour of your *lacks* as shown by the colour additions of your name vibration.

Black is a formal colour and gives dignity to the person and the occasion, but if too much black is worn it represents sorrow and loss. It tends to confine and repress the emotions, to close in the person, and does not attract others in true friendship and love. If black must be worn, a touch of colour should also be featured about the person.

Music in Healing

Every sound emits a certain colour and takes on definite form. We have seen this recently on television, where the colours emanating from the music have been shown on the television screen. Every form also gives forth a sound, which is its key-note. Every created thing, from a molecule to a man and from the planet to the solar system, possesses a key-note of its own. The sum total of these notes makes up the music of the spheres. Everything pulsates to a definite rhythm, including the universe itself as it circles the sun; the planets too have their notes.

Flowers, trees and grasses have their own symphonic sound. In fact a delicate instrument has been perfected in Germany whereby the sound of growing grass can be heard. The winds and the waves have their own rhythm and the combined rhythms make up the key-note of the planet. Likewise man's organs all emit their own notes and make up the key-note of the planet. Likewise man's organs all emit their own notes and make up the vital key-note of the individual. Max Heindel, a great German occultist, states that in health, the etheric body emits a sound which is like the hum of the bumble bee.

Since every object has its own key-note and overall blending of colours, it follows that upon entering a room one is immediately drawn to one person and repelled by another, often without a word being spoken. Where key-notes and colours harmonize there is understanding and affinity. Where they do not, the nerves are jarred and we say that so-and-so 'gets on my nerves'.

There are seven centres or *musical lights* which correspond with the seven chakras and the seven-toned musical scale.

Music helps to develop these centres progressively and enables them to unfold their powers, so that the chakras visible to clairvoyant sight emit beautiful colours as they rotate continuously. The first centre becomes a luminous red, the second a reddish orange becoming gradually shot through with a soft green light, the third or spleen centre becomes irradiated with a pure gold light, the fourth, the cardiac centre, emits a luminous yellow and ethereal blue light. The fifth (throat centre), an azure blue, gradually becomes shot through with silver as the centre develops. The sixth (brow centre), when fully developed, reveals the colours yellow, blue and purple forming patterns of beauty. The seventh centre, in the dome of the head, when the body has been fully regenerated, emits a pure white effulgent light which blesses all who come within its rays.

There are healers who work with music as well as colour and it has been demonstrated that an unbalanced mind is particularly sensitive to musical vibrations, so that restful music can soothe the most excitable and violent patients. Conversely it might be said that pop records would excite already unbalanced or violent people.

The healing value of music has been recognized from earliest times. For instance, Paracelsus, a seer and therapist prescribed certain compositions for certain maladies and practised Musical Healing. Today the power of discordant emotions to quickly or slowly destroy the physical body is much more understood, so that healing is not only directed at curing symptoms, but at reaching the seat of the disharmony in one of the subtle bodies, where such curative agents as music, colour, radionic treatment, homoeopathic medicaments and the Bach remedies, can heal the whole man.

So back to music itself and the fact that each one of us has a theme song which is formed from our names. Each number has its key-note on the musical scale.

Number	Letters	Key-note
1	A J S	middle C
2	B K T	D
3	C L U	E
4	D M V	F
5	E N W	G
6	F O X	A
7	G P Y	B
8	H Q Z	C (high C)
9	I R	D (high D)

Your 'Life Song'

If you understand music a little or are a musician, writing your 'life song' will cause you little trouble and in fact can be fascinating. You can use the chords of modern song writers to give it more charm. The numbers of the birthdate reduced to a single digit can be used to make a chorus. With each name a verse, the chorus can be the chords of the birthdate.

Your life song or musical key-note can be used to tune yourself to the purpose of your birth, and the playing of music which you enjoy and feel yourself attuned to can be the means of progressively unfolding the power of the centres or chakras. This tuning in to your 'life song' can be done either by singing or playing your key-note before meditation.

Frequent repetition of the chord of your own key-note can provide you with a wonderful system of protection against disease. It also has a soothing, harmonious effect on strained nerves or a tired body. The playing of this chord is also a wonderful way in which to lift the consciousness above the trials and difficulties of personal living and into the realms of inner knowing, where all is harmony and peace.

Astrological Applications

Those of you who are interested in astrology will like to know of the colour and musical correspondence inherent in your Sun sign and its relation to a particular part of the body. An illness is not always shown by the sign ruling the afflicted part. Sometimes it is shown equally well by the opposite sign, as the forces of the two signs intermingle in the body.

When the harmony of an organ of the body has been disrupted, disease is present until the rhythm and proper colour flow has been restored. The mind as a creative agent can heal the body, and to still the mind and quieten it so that it is better able to accomplish the healing of the physical body, it is best to play chords in the key of F and F sharp. The close affinity between opposite signs is shown by their musical relationship via their key-notes. *Virgo* and *Pisces*, for instance, have Virgo C and Pisces B for key-notes.

The key-note of *Aries* is D flat, the colour of *Aries* is red. In astrological terms it rules the head and so the ear, eye, nose and all cranial nerves. Spiritually, *Aries* releases the highest impulses of the spirit.

Libra is its opposite sign, its key-note is D natural and its colour blue. An harmonic based on D will therefore release a spiritual force for the healing of afflictions of the head or kidneys.

Taurus has the key-note E flat, ruling the throat and organs of speech. The colour related to Taurus is green. These organs are destined to become the seat of power in the human body.

The opposite sign to *Taurus* is *Scorpio*, which rules the organs of generation and so holds the mystery of creation; its key-note is E. A harmonic based on E will, therefore, release a spiritual force for the healing of afflictions affecting the throat, larynx or the generative organs. The colour of *Scorpio* is deep red.

Gemini's key-note is F sharp, and *Gemini* rules the lower mind and the lungs, the vital breath, arms and hands. The colour of *Gemini* is yellow.

Sagittarius is its opposite sign, and its key-note is F. It holds the pattern of the higher mind, though it awakens the spiritual power and aspiration which gives it sway over the lower material mind. A harmonic based on the key of F will release the spiritual force for the clearing of afflictions of the mind and of the lungs. The colour of *Sagittarius* is purple.

Cancer's key-note is G sharp, and it rules the stomach and the breasts; through it awakens the faculty of intuition. Its colour is silver.

Capricorn is its opposite sign and rules the

knees; its key-note is G, its colour black. This sign, using the key of G major, sends a ray of renewal to the earth. Therefore the key-note of *Cancer* is G sharp and that of *Capricorn* G natural. The key of G releases spiritual forces for the healing of diseases relating to the stomach, breasts and knees.

The key-note of *Leo* is A sharp and of its opposite sign – *Aquarius* – A natural. *Leo* rules the heart and the opposite polarity – *Aquarius* – the ankles and the circulation. The motivating power of *Leo* is love and of *Aquarius* mentality; their combination is said to be able to produce the superman of the Aquarian age. This is the union of heart and mind so difficult to achieve. The key of A releases spiritual forces for the healing of ills related to the heart, circulation and the ankles. The colour of *Leo* is gold and the colour of *Aquarius* blue.

The key-note of *Virgo* is C; *Virgo* rules the intestines and all their intricacies, its colour is brown, and its polarity is *Pisces*, whose sign rules the feet, the foundation of all understanding. The key-note of *Pisces* is B and its colour violet, its spiritual aim being the unity of all life. The keys of B and C major will release the spiritual forces for the healing of ills related to the intestines and the feet.

Sacred Temples

Colour and music work together to regenerate the body and these arts were used in the sacred temples of Egypt and Greece. Chants and invocations were spiritually constructed and so had powerful results. The priests taught the neophytes how to determine their key-notes, their sign and planet, and hereby gave them the ability to tune in on the power planetary. This wisdom and the use of colour, number and astrology, all formed part of the teaching of the Mysteries.

The Persians celebrated the entry of the Sun into each zodiacal sign with the appropriate chants and music, stressing the vibratory key-note of the zodiacal sign and its ruler.

Music is indeed not only a healing and regenerative influence, but also one which enables the gradual unfoldment of man's spiritual powers through the raising of the vibratory level of the body and the clearing and stimulating of the chakras.

CHAPTER SEVEN

GENERAL INFLUENCES OF COLOUR

Colour plays a big part in our lives. Nature provides us constantly with varied shades. A bright blue sky can lift our spirit and a dark cloudy sky can make us feel low and depressed. Sunshine brings joy to most of us. Each season of the year has different colour hues. I do not have to talk about them, you all have experienced them in your own way. When the sky is clear at night and the moon is full, some people are influenced by it favourably or unfavourably.

Everything has a certain frequency of vibration, and that applies to all organs in the human body. If there is any deviation from the normal vibrations, it shows that the organ is not functioning properly. All organs have a vibration of their own, and can be detected, and it is the healer's job to wipe out these disease vibrations of the body and restore them to normal health. The application of the right frequency will alter the faulty vibration and bring the organ back to normal. Fatigue, strain, stress, fear and all negative emotions are culprits upsetting the healthy vibrations. Colour being a pure vibration, when used in the right shade and focused on to the right place, can correct the fault and restore the body to health.

Colour can be visualized with some perseverance. One can use these colours for self-healing or one can send them out to patients. Then, of course, colour can be used with help of a colour lamp. In my own practice I use a De La Warr colourscope regularly.

There are 7 main colours in the spectrum: red, orange, yellow, green, blue. indigo and violet. The *warm colours* are *red, orange* and *yellow.*

Red is the element of fire and stimulates and excites the nerves and the blood. It releases adrenalin and stimulates the sensory nerves. It activates the circulation of the blood, excites the cerebro spinal nerves and the sympathetic nervous system. It vitalizes the physical body, but because it is such a great stimulant it must be used with caution. Over-stimulation can be dangerous. Health means balance.

Red is contra indicated in all inflammatory conditions and most emotional disturbances. One should never treat with red alone, but it should be followed either by green or blue.

Orange is a combination of red and yellow. It has an anti-spasmodic effect. It is good for the treatment of muscle-cramps and spasms. Orange aids the calcium metabolism and it strengthens the lungs, the pancreas and the spleen. This colour raises the pulse-rate, but it does not raise the blood-pressure. It releases energy from the spleen and the pancreas. Orange strengthens the etheric body, enlives the emotions and creates a general feeling of well-being, and cheerfulness.

Yellow activates the motor nerves. It generates energy in the muscle. It works favourably on the digestion, but if used for too long it might bring on diarrhoea, because it stimulates the flow of the bile. Yellow gets rid of parasites. It improves the skin and purifies the blood-stream. It activates the lymph. Yellow can depress the spleen. Psychologically it can get rid of melancholia and despondency. It is the colour of the intellect and of reason.

Yellow is contra indicated in acute inflammation, delirium diarrhoea, fever, over-excitement and palpitation of the heart.

Green is the middle colour of the spectrum. Green dilates the capillaries and produces a sensation of warmth. It relieves tension, but when used too much it gets tiring. It is a pituitary gland stimulant, and it is a muscle and tissue builder. Green is a disinfectant. Green loosens and at the same time regulates the etheric body and brings back the astral body which has suffered through shock, fatigue, illness or negative emotions.

Blue, indigo and violet are cooling colours.

Blue increases the metabolism. It promotes growth and suppuration. It heals burns very quickly. Blue is the colour of intuition and higher mental faculties.

Blue is contra-indicated for colds, gout, hypertension, muscle contractions, paralysis, chronic rheumatism and tachycardia (rapid heartbeat.)

Indigo is cooling, astringent, and electric. It works on the parathyroid glands, but depresses the thyroids. So when the thyroid is overworking, one treats the parathyroids with indigo. It purifies the blood-stream, and builds phagocites in the spleen. It reduces or even stops bleeding. When excessive bleeding is present, always treat the parathyroids with indigo. It depresses the respiration and is good for muscle toning. It has an anaesthetic effect when used too long. Indigo affects the vision, hearing and smell. It also affects the emotional and spiritual levels, and mental complaints with delirium tremens and insanity. One can get rid of obsessions with it, but in the latter case the healer has to protect himself or herself as the case may be, not to pick the obsession up.

Violet depresses the motor nerves and the lymphatic system, as well as the cardiac system. It purifies the blood and is a leucocyte builder. Violet maintains the potassium balance in the body. It stops the growth of tumours. When treating cancer patients after they have had their operation three colours help:

Red to give energy to the system.

Green to stabilize the astral body.

Violet to restore the potassium-sodium balance.

Violet is a good and calming colour in cases of violent insanity. It controls excess hunger. It is a spiritual colour. The power of meditation is much deeper under violet light. The Compte Saint Germaine healed mostly with violet rays.

Ultra-violet is beyond the visible spectrum. It plays a very important part in the calcium-phosphorous metabolism. It fixes iron and iodine, therefore it is useful in the treatment of goitres and rickets. It normalizes the metabolism and glandular activities. It stimulates the action of the sympathetic nervous system and helps to ease pain. It acts favourably on the heart and on the lungs. There are combinations of shades which used in colour treatment:

Lemon which is a mixture of a very light yellow and a very light green. Lemon rejuvenates the organism and throws out toxins. It is a laxative, eliminates phlegm, and strengthens the bones. It is a cerebral stimulant, activates the thymus gland, cures cretinism. It is antacid.

Purple and *Scarlet* which are combinations of red and blue. Purple is more blue and less red. Scarlet is more red and less blue.

Purple has an analgesic property. It suppresses malaria, and it is a venous stimulant.

Scarlet stimulates the kidneys and the sexual mechanism.

Magenta is a combination of red and violet and it energizes the adrenal glands and the action of the heart. It is a diuretic. In some cases it is an emotional stabilizer.

Turquoise is the opposite of the lemon ray. Builds the skin. When a burn is treated with blue, it might help to use the turquoise afterwards to hasten the skin formation. It is a cerebral depressant. It lowers mental over-activity.

Complementary Colours
Each colour has a complementary colour.

Red	—	Blue
Orange	—	Violet
Yellow	—	Violet
Green	—	Magenta
Blue	—	Red
Indigo	—	Orange
Violet	—	Yellow

   Those who use the pendulum are at an advantage with regard to diagnosing and colour selectivity and duration of treatment. Patients should not only be treated for the illness they complain of, but they should be treated on three levels. For the illness on the physical level, then on the etheric level, which comprises the nervous system and on the astral which comprises the ductless glands and the emotions. When one looks at the aura, most people can only see the vibrations of the just mentioned 3 bodies, but it is difficult to see the vibrations of the higher developed bodies. In the aura the physical vibration is always in a fixed position very near to the physical body. The etheric vibration is more or less always in a near proximity, though it can look congested or as a double of the physical one, when it is in good health. The astral sheath is movable. It can be like a third layer, in a normal position, round the etheric, or it can be away from the body. In shock or emotional disturbances it moves from its normal position. After an operation the practitioner must first remove the anaesthetic toxins and then attend to the astral body.

Colour Vibrations of Some Foods

Red, orange and *yellow* foods have an alkaline effect.

Green foods are neither acid nor alkaline, they are neutral.

Blue, indigo and *violet* foods have an acid effect.

Red foods:	meat, all red skinned fruits and vegetables, watercress, beets, cabbage, cherries, peppers, grapes, onions, radishes.
Orange foods:	carrots, oranges, pumpkins, sweet corn, apricots, tangerines and peaches.
Yellow foods:	apricots, butter, egg yolks, carrots, sweet corn, grapefruits, mangoes, melons, marrow and yellow skinned fruits and vegetables.
Green foods:	green vegetables and fruits of that colour.
Blue foods:	most blue fruits like plums, blueberries, bilberries, fish, veal, asparagus, potatoes.
Indigo foods:	these are the same as the blue and violet foods.
Violet foods:	aubergines, purple broccoli, beet, purple grapes and blackberries.

Colour in the Home

When you plan to decorate a room think whether you want the room to look bigger or smaller.

Red, orange and *yellow* make a room look smaller, while

White, blue and *indigo* make a room look larger.

Green keeps it in the right proportion.

Blue draws the ego and brings harmony with the environment. It brings the introvert out of his shell.

Red makes a person egocentric, and *green* is very good on the cardiac circulation.

Colours of the Ductless Glands

So far only colours from the health angle were mentioned. Now let us look into the colours of the ductless glands in relation to the planetary influence. If we consider the spiritual connection of the ductless glands with the latent potentialities, we find that they need different colours and much lighter shades. The spiritual colours of the glands are:

Dazzling blue	—	Pineal gland
Light yellow	—	Pituitary gland
Violet	—	Thyroid gland
Light golden yellow	—	Thymus gland
Golden yellow	—	Spleen
Blue	—	Adrenal glands

The Adrenals are ruled by Jupiter.

When well aspected:

benevolence,
vision,
optimism,
courtesy,
generosity,
cheerfulness,
religious understanding

When badly aspected:

over-confidence
extravagance
conceit
lawlessness
procrastination

The Spleen is ruled by the Sun.

When well aspected:

vitality
courage
generosity
dignity
loyalty
faithfulness
parental instinct
leadership
responsibility

When badly aspected:

arrogance
overbearing and a domineering nature

The Thymus gland is under the love ray of
Venus.

When well aspected:

The individual develops the highest form of
love
artistic ability
sense of beauty
cheerfulness
charm

When badly aspected:

sensuality
vulgarity
sentimentality
vanity
inconsistency

The Thyroid gland is under the rulership of
Mercury.

When well aspected:

dexterity
reason
intellect
thoughtfulness
good memory
studiousness
quick wit
eloquence

When badly aspected:

conceit
cunning
carelessness
lack of principles
gossiping
dishonesty
gambling
indecision
nervousness

The Pituitary Gland is under the rulership of Uranus.

When well aspected:

originality
love of liberty for all
independence
reformation
progression
intuition
mysticism
(when in good harmony with a well aspected Pineal, clairvoyance.)

When badly aspected:

eccentricity
fanaticism
irresponsibility
perversion
impatience
(and in some cases, anarchy.)

The Pituitary body is the spiritual chain which connects Man with the highest vibrations of the Christ Spirit. The primary seat of this gland is the life spirit and the heart is the secondary seat. The colour of the life spirit is yellow. The Pituitary is closely connected with the mystic path which leads to perfect Initiation. The arousing of the Pituitary body into action is one of the most important accomplishments in the development of the powers of the spirit.

The Pineal body is ruled by *Neptune*. The spiritual side of the Pineal rules Neptune, but on the intellectual level, Mercury. When Neptune is not well aspected the individual does not only deceive others, but himself as well.

When well aspected:

contact with the super physical
inspiration
clairvoyance
prophecy
devotion
occultism
divinity
philosophy

When badly aspected:

delusion
morbidity
unreality
obsession
intrigue
black magic
a chaotic mental condition.

This does not mean to say that all the mentioned traits are in each individual, but some of them are in all of us.

The Spiritual Side of Man is represented by the *Pituitary and the Pineal glands*.

The Personality by the *Adrenals* and the *Thymus*, and *the link between them* is the *Thyroid gland*. It is much easier to improve on the physical vibrations and on the emotional ones, than on the spiritual ones. Not only desire of the individual is necessary, but the person's Karma also has to be considered. If the person in question can visualize the colour, the improvement is quicker, than when it is sent out.

INDEX